SIMPLIFIED GUIDE ON

HAWAIIAN LOMI LOMI MASSAGE

Discover The Essence Of Aloha Spirit In Healing Body, Mind, And Soul With Traditional Lomi Lomi Practices

DR. ARIYA REYNA

CONTENTS

Copyright © 2023, By Dr. Ariya Reyna

All Rights Reserved

DISCLIAMER

This book is intended for informational purposes only and is not a substitute for professional medical advice, diagnosis, or treatment. The information provided in this book is based on the author's research and personal experiences and is not meant to replace the advice of healthcare professionals.

Readers are encouraged to consult with their healthcare providers before beginning any new exercise, wellness, or health program.

The author and publisher of this book are not responsible for any specific health or allergy needs that may require medical supervision and are not liable for any damages or negative consequences from any treatment, action, application, or preparation, to any person reading or following the information in this book.

The content of this book is not intended to be a substitute for professional medical advice, diagnosis, or treatment. Always seek the advice of your physician or other qualified health provider with any questions you may have regarding a medical condition.

The author and publisher disclaim responsibility for any adverse effects that may result from the use or application of the information contained in this book.

References to specific products, services, or organizations do not imply endorsement or recommendation by the author or the publisher.

The inclusion of such references is for illustrative purposes only. Thank you for reading and respecting the terms outlined in this disclaimer.

CHAPTER ONE

An Overview Of Hawaiian Lomi Lomi Massage

Hawaiian Lomi Lomi massage is a traditional Polynesian healing technique with profound roots in Hawaiian culture and spirituality. Lomi Lomi massage, also known as "Loving Hands" massage, is a holistic approach to wellbeing that extends beyond the physical components of massage. It is a holy and ceremonial activity that includes spiritual, mental, and physical healing as well as physical relaxation.

Historical Origins And Cultural Importance

To comprehend Hawaiian Lomi Lomi massage, one must first learn about its historical origins and cultural relevance. The technique derives from the Hawaiian Islands' historic healing practices, which were passed down through generations within families. Lomi Lomi was more than simply a massage method for the Hawaiians; it was a way of life. The technique was firmly embedded in the culture, expressing the spiritual link between the healer, the receiver, and the natural forces surrounding them.

Historically, native healers, or "kahuna alpacas," employed Lomi Lomi to promote physical and spiritual well-being in their communities. To boost the therapeutic energy, the massage was frequently given in sacred settings like temples or outdoors surrounded by nature. Lomi Lomi has cultural importance beyond the massage table, symbolizing a holistic approach to wellness that includes the mind, body, and spirit.

The Lomi Lomi Philosophical Foundation

A distinct and profound concept distinguishes Hawaiian Lomi Lomi massage from other massage styles. The term "pono," which in Hawaiian means "righteousness" or "balance," is the source of the concept. Lomi Lomi strives to restore body and soul balance and harmony, acknowledging that physical diseases can have spiritual or emotional bases.

The technique is founded on the notion that the body contains memories and emotions that may be released and healed through the art of touch. Lomi Lomi practitioners see the body as a whole, knowing that emotional and mental well-being are inextricably linked to physical health. Lomi Lomi seeks to induce not just relaxation but also emotional release and spiritual healing by treating the body as a whole.

Traditional Hawaiian Healing Concepts

Hawaiian Lomi Lomi massage combines ancient Hawaiian healing principles, stressing the individual's oneness with nature and the divine. The Hawaiian worldview, known as "Huna," acknowledges that all living things are linked by a divine force. Lomi Lomi practitioners direct this energy to aid in healing.

The belief in "mana," the life force or spiritual energy that runs through all living things, is a critical component. To facilitate healing, the practitioner channels their mana and connects with the client's mana in Lomi Lomi. This link is said to be necessary for energy to flow freely, resulting in bodily and spiritual harmony.

Another crucial notion is "aloha," which extends beyond a basic welcome. Aloha represents love, compassion, and a great regard for others. Lomi Lomi practitioners integrate aloha into their massages, creating a compassionate and comfortable environment for healing to take place. This emphasis on love and compassion leads to Lomi Lomi Massage's unique and transforming character.

Techniques For Lomi Lomi Massage

Hawaiian Lomi Lomi massage techniques are as distinct as its philosophy. Hands, forearms, and elbows are used to produce fluid, rhythmic strokes that simulate the ebb and flow of the ocean. Long, continuous strokes are used to induce relaxation, relieve tension, and increase energy flow throughout the body.

Forearm runs, in which the practitioner's forearms glide over the recipient's body in lengthy, sweeping strokes, are one distinguishing feature of Lomi Lomi. This method applies wide and even pressure to huge portions of the body, giving a sensation of oneness among the various components. The constant flow of strokes is thought to promote the discharge of physical and mental barriers.

Stretching and joint mobilization are also frequent in Lomi Lomi, enhancing flexibility and relieving stress. To improve the whole experience, the practitioner may use light rocking or swaying movements. These techniques add to the massage's comprehensive character by treating both the physical and energetic components of the individual.

In Lomi Lomi massage, the practitioner's purpose and presence are as important as the physical techniques. Massage is a spiritual dance between the provider and receiver governed by the ideals of aloha and pono.

The practitioner's energy and purpose are important in supporting tension release and generating a sense of well-being.

To summarize, Hawaiian Lomi Lomi massage is more than a treatment; it is a cultural and spiritual practice strongly steeped in Hawaiian traditions. Its philosophy, which is based on the ideals of balance, connectivity, and love, distinguishes it as a holistic approach to healing. The methods, which are distinguished by flowing and rhythmic strokes, are intended to restore balance to the body, mind, and spirit. Lomi Lomi delivers a transforming experience that goes beyond the physical sphere, offering a space for healing on various levels as a unique combination of tradition, philosophy, and touch.

Lomi Lomi Massage Movements And Strokes

Hawaiian Lomi Lomi massage, often known as "the loving hand's massage," is a traditional Polynesian therapeutic therapy with distinctive strokes and motions.

Lomi Lomi extends beyond the physical side of massage, trying to restore harmony and balance to the body, mind, and spirit. It is based on the traditional knowledge of the Hawaiian people.

The use of continuous, flowing strokes that mirror the movement of ocean waves is a distinguishing element of Lomi Lomi. Therapists utilize their hands, forearms, and even elbows to move across the recipient's body in a dance-like motion. Not only are the rhythmic and flowing strokes physically calming, but they also strive to clear emotional and energy blocks.

Lomi Lomi strokes are intended to mirror the ebb and flow of life, representing the interconnection of all things. Long, sweeping strokes that cross the full length of the body may be used by the therapist to promote a sense of togetherness and oneness. Circular and figure-eight motions are also frequent, symbolizing life's cyclical cycle and the constant flow of energy.

Lomi Lomi incorporates joint rotations and stretches in addition to physical strokes. These motions aid in flexibility, tension release, and total range of motion. The therapist may lead the client through mild stretches to promote openness and allow the body to release stored tension.

Lomi Lomi massage strokes are profoundly anchored in the therapist's purpose as much as the mechanics of touch. The practitioner's concentration on love, compassion, and healing energy is said to enhance the massage's therapeutic benefits, making it a holistic and transforming experience.

CHAPTER TWO

The Role Of Intention And Breath In Lomi Lomi

The notion that the breath is a potent energy that connects the physical and spiritual realms is central to the Lomi Lomi massage philosophy. Conscious breathing is emphasized by practitioners as a technique for facilitating the free passage of energy and enhancing the therapeutic effects of massage.

Throughout the therapy, both the therapist and the receiver are urged to take deep, synchronized breaths. This deliberate breathing not only improves relaxation but also acts as a channel for energy exchange. The rhythmic inhales and exhales form a perfect dance, bringing the energies of the provider and receiver into alignment.

Another important part of Lomi Lomi is the intention, which goes hand in hand with conscious breathing. The therapist sets a good and therapeutic intention for the massage session before it begins.

This goal serves as a guiding force, instilling a sense of purpose in the massage that goes beyond the actual manipulation of muscles. To develop a collaborative and co-creative healing process, the recipient is also urged to establish their intentions.

In Lomi Lomi, the combination of breath and intention produces a holy and transforming atmosphere. Massage becomes a comprehensive experience as the therapist's hands move with the rhythm of the breath and the force of purpose, addressing not just the person's physical body but also their emotional and spiritual aspects.

Ceremonies And Rituals Of Lomi Lomi

Lomi Lomi massage is more than just a spa treatment; it is frequently seen as a holy ritual and ceremonial. Lomi Lomi, which is rooted in Hawaii's rich cultural and spiritual traditions, is considered a method to honor and connect with the divine, nature, and one's ancestors.

A Lomi Lomi session is frequently preceded by a ceremonial opening in which the therapist gives a prayer or chant to evoke positive energies and create a holy atmosphere. This ceremonial technique sets the tone for the massage, transforming it into a profoundly spiritual experience.

To enhance the ceremonial ambiance, practitioners may use traditional Hawaiian music, chanting, or the sound of ocean waves throughout the massage. The utilization of these audio elements is said to resonate with the natural rhythms of the body and the Earth, enhancing the massage's therapeutic energy.

The inclusion of symbolism and religious gestures is another important part of Lomi Lomi rites. During the session, the therapist may employ symbolic materials such as feathers, shells, or crystals, infusing them with specific goals and energy. These artifacts were picked for their spiritual significance and are said to transmit natural healing energy.

The end of a Lomi Lomi session is just as ceremonial as the beginning. The therapist may conclude with a prayer or blessing, expressing thanks for the healing that has occurred. This conclusion is an important aspect of the ritual because it ensures that the receiver exits the session feeling not only physically relaxed but also spiritually nourished.

Massage Oils And Tools For Lomi Lomi

Massage oils and instruments are used in Lomi Lomi to enhance the entire experience and therapeutic effects. Coconut oil, a traditional Hawaiian oil, is widely utilized for its nourishing and moisturizing characteristics. The aroma of these oils provides another dimension to the sensory experience, helping to the recipient's relaxation and grounding.

The oils used in Lomi Lomi are chosen not only for their physical properties, but also for their symbolic and spiritual value. For example, coconut oil is regarded as a sign of purity and is said to contain the essence of a tropical paradise. This is consistent with the wider Lomi Lomi worldview, which attempts to link the individual with the natural environment and its healing forces.

In addition to oils, therapists in Lomi Lomi may utilize other instruments to improve the massage experience. Hot stones, for example, can be used to offer a calming and anchoring effect. The warmth of the stones aids in muscular relaxation, allowing for a deeper release of tension. Stones are also associated with the elemental and earth-centered parts of Hawaiian spirituality.

Natural things such as feathers, shells, and other natural objects can be utilized as extensions of the therapist's hands, providing a distinct and tactile touch to the massage. These instruments are chosen for their spiritual importance, signifying the relationship between the human body and the natural world, rather than their practical use.

The Advantages Of Hawaiian Lomi Lomi Massage

Hawaiian Lomi Lomi massage has several physical, mental, and spiritual advantages, making it a comprehensive approach to well-being. The one-of-a-kind combination of flowing strokes, purposeful breathwork, and ceremonial aspects combines to a transforming experience for both provider and recipient.

Lomi Lomi helps to relieve stress, improve circulation, and increase flexibility. The rhythmic strokes and joint motions reduce muscular tightness and develop physical equilibrium. Massage oils and instruments give an added layer of sensory enjoyment, adding to full body relaxation.

Lomi Lomi provides a secure and supportive environment for people to release tension, anxiety, and emotional blocks. The therapist's loving intention, along with the constant flow of strokes, produces an environment that facilitates emotional release and inner serenity.

Following a Lomi Lomi session, many recipients report a tremendous sensation of relaxation and emotional clarity.

Lomi Lomi massage links people with the deepest components of their being and the world around them spiritually.

Massage is elevated to a spiritual experience by including breath, intention, and ceremonial aspects. It allows for spiritual meditation, alignment, and a connection with the natural forces that control existence.

Lomi Lomi's collaborative character, in which both the therapist and the receiver actively participate in the healing process, promotes a sense of togetherness and connectivity. Because of this comprehensive approach to well-being, Lomi Lomi is more than simply a massage; it is a transforming experience that embraces the body, mind, and soul.

Including Spirituality In Lomi Lomi

Hawaiian Lomi Lomi massage is more than simply physical rehabilitation; it is a comprehensive method with spirituality at its heart. Lomi Lomi, which is based on the ancient Hawaiian concept of Huna, goes beyond the manipulation of muscles and tissues to aim to balance the body, mind, and spirit. The spiritual part of Lomi Lomi is firmly ingrained in the ancient practice and is said to be crucial for general well-being.

The practitioner of Lomi Lomi frequently opens the session with a prayer or blessing, stating the goal for healing and seeking spiritual help. This ceremony is intended to create a holy place in which both the giver and the recipient can connect with divine energy.

Massage strokes, often known as "dance of the hands," are more than simply physical motions; they are a type of energy communication aimed at restoring balance and harmony to the recipient's complete body.

Lomi Lomi is founded on the notion of 'aloha,' often known as the Hawaiian spirit of love, compassion, and connection.

Practitioners believe that by bringing love and positive energy into their touch, they may help the body release stress and bad emotions. This spiritual link is thought to be crucial in releasing the body's innate potential to repair itself.

Furthermore, Lomi Lomi massage promotes submission and confidence in the healing process. This submission extends beyond the bodily to a deeper, spiritual level. It is thought that as the message develops, the recipient's spirit gets more linked with the universal life force, generating a sense of inner calm and tranquillity.

While the spiritual side of Lomi Lomi is not openly religious, it is strongly anchored in Hawaii's cultural and spiritual traditions. Massage therapists are frequently educated not just in massage methods, but also in the cultural and spiritual factors that support the profession.

This assures that the essence of Lomi Lomi is kept and passed down through generations, including its spiritual elements.

CHAPTER THREE

Lomi Lomi Training And Certification

Lomi Lomi massage is a specialist style of bodywork that necessitates a distinct set of skills and knowledge. Training and certification in Lomi Lomi are essential not only for assuring competent massage delivery but also for preserving the cultural integrity and spiritual dimensions of the practice.

Formal Lomi Lomi training often includes themes such as the practice's history and philosophy, anatomy and physiology, particular massage methods, and cultural sensitivity.

Many training programs also highlight Lomi Lomi's spiritual components, teaching practitioners how to include intention, breathwork, and energy connection in their sessions.

Lomi Lomi certification is frequently gained through recognized colleges and training institutes that specialize in Hawaiian healing arts. These programs can range in length from brief seminars to longer courses lasting many months. Some programs may even incorporate a cultural immersion component to help practitioners better comprehend the spiritual and cultural backdrop of Lomi Lomi.

In addition to formal training, many Lomi Lomi practitioners pursue continuing professional development and seek mentorship from experienced instructors. This dedication to lifelong study is vital for remaining linked to the shifting traditions of Lomi Lomi and enhancing one's talents throughout time.

Certification not only certifies a practitioner's skill, but it also acts as a symbol of cultural understanding and respect. It shows that the practitioner has received sufficient training and knows the significance of maintaining the integrity of Lomi Lomi. Clients may trust the practitioner to provide a massage that is not only physically helpful but also culturally and spiritually appropriate.

Modern Lomi Lomi Massage Applications

Lomi Lomi massage, while strongly steeped in ancient Hawaiian traditions, has made its way into current health practices and massage treatment. Lomi Lomi's versatility stems from its holistic approach, which addresses both the physical and spiritual components of well-being.

Lomi Lomi is frequently given as a delightful and revitalizing massage experience in modern spa settings. The use of forearms and long, flowing strokes generate a sensation of fluidity that separates Lomi Lomi from other massage treatments. This distinctive approach has grown in popularity because of its capacity to produce relaxation and alleviate tension, making it a sought-after therapy in today's fast-paced environment.

Lomi Lomi has been used in holistic health practices, wellness retreats, and alternative medical techniques in addition to its use in spas.

To increase the therapeutic effects of Lomi Lomi, some practitioners mix it with additional treatments such as energy healing or aromatherapy. Lomi Lomi's versatility allows it to supplement diverse wellness techniques, making it a flexible tool for holistic health practitioners.

Lomi Lomi's emphasis on restoring balance and harmony makes it a viable addition to standard treatment procedures in rehabilitation and physical therapy settings. The mild yet effective procedures may be modified to address individual musculoskeletal concerns while also developing flexibility and relieving stress.

Furthermore, the spiritual components of Lomi Lomi make it appealing to those seeking a deeper connection with their body and spirit. Lomi Lomi is revered in mindfulness and meditation circles for its capacity to produce a contemplative state, assisting individuals in releasing mental and emotional blocks.

As Lomi Lomi evolves and adapts to meet the requirements of the modern world, its essential concepts of love, connection, and holistic healing remain central to its current applications.

Cultural Awareness And Respect In Lomi Lomi Practice

Cultural sensitivity and respect are fundamental values in Lomi Lomi massage therapy. Lomi Lomi is an ancient Hawaiian healing technique that is profoundly entwined with the Hawaiian people's cultural and spiritual heritage. Practitioners are educated not just in physical methods, but also in the cultural framework that gives the practice significance.

Respect for Lomi Lomi's cultural background is clear from the start of the session. Practitioners frequently begin with a traditional opening, which may include a prayer or chant to establish a reverent tone and connect with the spiritual parts of the practice. This cultural acknowledgment is more than simply a formality; it is critical to the integrity of Lomi Lomi.

Additionally, Lomi Lomi practitioners are expected to embody the spirit of 'aloha' during the practice. This entails injecting love, compassion, and positive energy into their touch. The goal of each stroke is to build a therapeutic connection that extends beyond the physical body, not just to manipulate muscles.

Lomi Lomi cultural awareness extends to the use of language, symbolism, and traditional components in the practice. Practitioners are conscious of the importance of certain phrases, gestures, or instruments, ensuring that their use is consistent with Hawaiian cultural traditions. This attention to cultural detail is critical for preventing cultural appropriation and preserving Lomi Lomi's originality.

Furthermore, practitioners frequently participate in cultural immersion activities to increase their awareness of Hawaiian customs.

Learning about the history of the islands, engaging in traditional rites, and having a true respect for the rich cultural fabric that informs Lomi Lomi are all examples of this.

Clients, too, contribute to cultural awareness during a Lomi Lomi session. They are advised to approach the activity with an open mind and openness to the cultural background. Understanding and honoring Lomi Lomi's spiritual and cultural components enriches the whole experience and helps to a deeper feeling of healing.

Client Preparation And Follow-Up

Client preparation and aftercare are essential components of the Lomi Lomi experience, and they contribute to the overall efficacy and durability of the massage effects. Proper preparation and post-massage care are critical for enhancing the session's physical, emotional, and spiritual effects.

Clients are frequently instructed to establish an aim for their session before the massage begins. The purpose of this intention-setting ritual is to link the client's goals with the therapeutic aims of Lomi Lomi. Clarifying the aim, whether for relaxation, stress alleviation, or physical healing, provides a focused and purposeful setting for the session.

Clients may be instructed to remove jewelry, wear comfortable clothes, and indicate any specific areas of concern or discomfort. This allows the practitioner to personalize the massage to the client's specific requirements while also establishing a secure and comfortable atmosphere.

Clients are asked to submit to the experience during the massage, allowing the practitioner's motions to aid the release of tension and energy blockages. The greater the client's openness and receptivity, the more powerful the influence of Lomi Lomi on both the physical and spiritual levels.

Following the session, practitioners frequently offer advice on post-massage care. This may include water, rest, and modest exercise recommendations to aid the body's natural healing process. Clients are encouraged to listen to their bodies, pay attention to any feelings or emotions that occur, and allow time for the healing experience to integrate.

Hydration is especially important since Lomi Lomi is thought to promote the body's natural detoxifying mechanisms. Drinking water aids in the removal of toxins from the body, hence improving general health. Clients may also be encouraged to engage in relaxing activities such as taking a warm bath, practicing deep breathing, or spending time in nature.

It is critical for good aftercare that the client and practitioner maintain an open channel of contact. Clients are frequently asked to share their experiences, ask questions, and seek further self-care support. This collaborative approach broadens the client's awareness of Lomi Lomi's comprehensive nature and encourages them to actively engage in their well-being.

Finally, client preparation and aftercare in Lomi Lomi go beyond the physical parts of the massage to include emotional and spiritual aspects. Lomi Lomi practitioners and clients contribute to a holistic and transformational healing experience by integrating intention-setting, physical preparation, and mindful aftercare.

CHAPTER FOUR

Popular Lomi Lomi Massage Variations

Hawaiian Lomi Lomi massage is a traditional therapeutic therapy that is strongly established in Hawaiian culture. Lomi Lomi is more than simply a massage; it is a comprehensive approach to treating the body, mind, and soul. It is known for its rhythmic and flowing motions. Various types and interpretations of Lomi Lomi have arisen throughout the years, each with its distinct qualities and therapeutic advantages.

The "Temple Style" or "Lomi Ha" is a popular form of Lomi Lomi that typically integrates traditional Hawaiian ceremonies and chants, producing a ceremonial and spiritually profound experience. Temple Style Lomi Lomi practitioners believe that the energy and purpose underlying the massage are critical to its success in bringing healing and balance.

Another prominent variety is the "Big Island Style," also known as "Lomi Ale Ale," which is distinguished by a more aggressive and deep tissue technique, with strong strokes aimed at releasing tension and promoting muscular relaxation. Individuals seeking a more intensive massage treatment to address particular physical ailments frequently use Lomi Ale Ale.

The "Heartworks Lomi" technique, on the other hand, concentrates on emotional and spiritual healing. Practitioners of this approach believe that the heart is the center of one's well-being and that emotional blockages may be freed via loving touch and focused movement.

Heartworks Lomi employs soft yet strong strokes to provide a compassionate and supportive atmosphere for emotional release and healing.

Each Lomi Lomi massage variety represents the many viewpoints within Hawaiian culture, emphasizing the importance of individual preferences and requirements. Clients can select a style according to their intended results, such as bodily alleviation, spiritual connection, or emotional recovery.

Success Stories And Case Studies

Lomi Lomi massage has grown in popularity due to its unique techniques as well as its ability to address a wide spectrum of physical and mental disorders. Numerous case studies and success stories demonstrate how this ancient Hawaiian method may improve lives.

One noteworthy case study includes a person who had persistent back pain and restricted mobility.

The client saw remarkable improvement in both pain levels and range of motion after a series of Lomi Lomi sessions. The flowing and rhythmic strokes of Lomi Lomi assisted in the release of muscular tension, encouraging relaxation and greater flexibility.

Another success story is a customer who sought the therapeutic advantages of Lomi Lomi massage due to stress and anxiety. The practitioner used soft yet careful strokes to create a peaceful and supportive environment for the client. The customer reported lower stress, increased sleep, and a general sense of well-being after numerous sessions.

These case studies show how Lomi Lomi massage may be used to heal both physical and emotional issues. Lomi Lomi's holistic approach, which takes into account the interdependence of the body, mind, and spirit, adds to its success in facilitating healing on numerous levels.

Considerations And Obstacles In Lomi Lomi Practice

While Lomi Lomi massage has significant advantages, practitioners must deal with obstacles and issues that are specific to this ancient Hawaiian therapy. One problem is maintaining cultural authenticity. As Lomi Lomi becomes more famous across the world, there is a possibility of theft or commercialization, which might dilute the holy and spiritual qualities of the practice.

Practitioners must strike a balance between presenting this ancient art form with a wider audience and preserving Lomi Lomi's cultural integrity. Respecting the spiritual chants, rituals, and cultural background that are frequently intermingled with the massage experience is part of this.

Another factor to consider is the requirement for continual education and skill development. Lomi Lomi is a fluid exercise with many different forms and interpretations. Practitioners must keep current on new techniques and continue to hone their abilities to satisfy the unique demands of their customers. Understanding the cultural subtleties and significance of certain practices is also essential for creating a genuine Lomi Lomi experience.

The physical demands of Lomi Lomi massage can often be difficult for practitioners.

To minimize fatigue or injury, the rhythmic and flowing motions need stamina and appropriate body mechanics. Regular self-care activities, such as receiving Lomi Lomi from fellow practitioners, can help practitioners maintain their well-being.

Lomi Lomi Massage Ethical Standards

Maintaining strong ethical standards is critical in Lomi Lomi massage therapy. As a traditional healing art profoundly established in Hawaiian culture, practitioners are charged with safeguarding the practice's integrity and valuing their customers' well-being.

In terms of informed consent, Lomi Lomi practitioners must communicate openly with their customers, describing the nature of the message, its potential benefits, and any potential discomfort or emotional release. Establishing trust and open communication is critical for clients to feel powerful and at ease throughout the session.

Another crucial part of ethical conduct in Lomi Lomi is cultural sensitivity. Practitioners must be aware of the cultural background and meaning of certain practices, chants, and rituals. To have a better grasp of the traditional characteristics of Lomi Lomi, it is critical to prevent appropriation and to seek help from cultural specialists or elders.

Maintaining customer privacy and confidence requires strict confidentiality. Practitioners must guarantee that all client information, whether verbal or written, is treated with care and not shared without specific agreement. This dedication to anonymity adds to the overall sense of safety and security that clients should have throughout a Lomi Lomi session.

Furthermore, practitioners must be aware of the power dynamics that exist in the client-practitioner interaction. It is critical to establish clear limits and maintain a professional manner to foster a safe and courteous atmosphere. Practitioners must be mindful of their intents and prejudices to keep the focus on the client's well-being rather than personal ambitions.

Finally, with its rich cultural origins and therapeutic advantages, Lomi Lomi massage has evolved into a variety of techniques and uses. Case studies and success stories demonstrate its usefulness in dealing with physical and mental issues. Practitioners, on the other hand, must deal with issues such as cultural preservation, continual education, and physical demands. Maintaining ethical standards is critical to ensuring that Lomi Lomi continues to be a respectful and transformational healing experience for everybody.

Conclusion

Finally, Hawaiian lomi lomi massage provides a highly refreshing and spiritually enlightening experience that transcends the physical sphere. This therapeutic technique, rooted in ancient Hawaiian traditions, harmonizes the body, mind, and spirit via rhythmic movements, purposeful contact, and the infusion of aloha, the spirit of love and compassion.

Tension evaporates and energy blockages are release as the massage therapist's hands dance gently across the body, promoting a profound sensation of relaxation and well-being.

The lomi lomi massage is more than just a kind of physical treatment; it is a holistic experience that reconnects people to the spirit of aloha and the natural flow of life.

A lomi lomi treatment concludes with a profound quiet, leaving recipients in a state of joyful tranquility. Clients frequently experience increased awareness, better circulation, and a restored sense of balance. Aside from the physiological advantages, the massage has a spiritual component that fosters a connection to the ancient knowledge rooted in Hawaiian culture.

In essence, the ultimate result of a Hawaiian lomi lomi massage transcends the treatment room, providing a ripple effect of good energy and overall well-being that can be felt in one's everyday life.

It is a time-honored practice that goes beyond the confines of traditional massage, providing a one-of-a-kind and transforming experience for people seeking not just physical comfort but also a deeper connection to the spirit of aloha.

THE END